Expecting In Shape

Nutrition for a Healthy Pregnancy Fueling Your Body and Baby

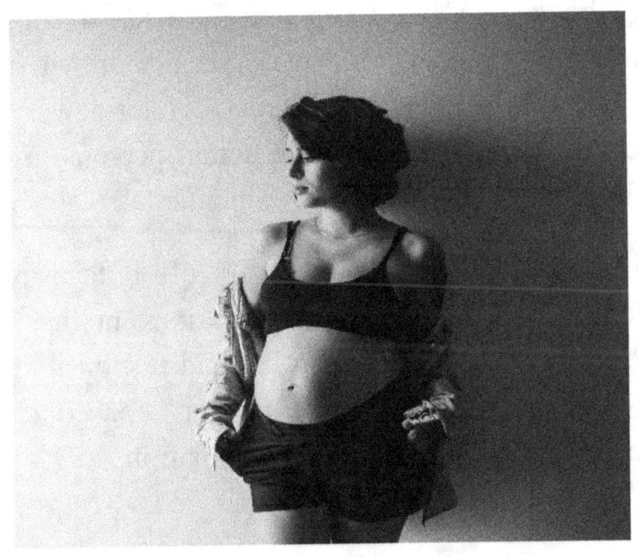

Thomas P. Tinney

Copyright © [2023] by [Thomas P. Tinney]

This book is a work of non-fiction. All of the characters, incidents, and dialogue are drawn from the author's personal experiences, interviews, and research. Any resemblance to actual persons, living or dead, or events is entirely coincidental.

While the author has made every effort to provide accurate and up-to-date information, neither the author nor the publisher can be held responsible for any errors or omissions or for any consequences resulting from the use of this information.

Contents

Chapter One

1.0 Introductory

Mamali had always been active, but when she discovered she had her first kid, she wasn't entirely sure how to keep her workout regimen safe. She didn't want to give up her health practices just because she was pregnant, but she didn't want to take any extra risks.

Thus, Mamali decided to educate herself on exercising correctly during pregnancy. She stumbled and discovered a book, "Expecting in Shape, "which explained all she needed to know about being active while pregnant.

Eager to learn more, Mamali went into the book and realized that exercising during pregnancy was safe and advantageous for both her and her baby's health. She read about the numerous sorts of workouts she might perform, such as walking, swimming, and prenatal yoga, as well as the necessity of good hydration and nutrition.

Mamali started adding these exercises to her regular regimen and realized she had more energy and less nervousness. She also discovered that exercise helped ease typical pregnancy discomforts, such as back pain and edema.

As she concluded her pregnancy, Mamali concentrated on activities preparing her for labor and delivery, such as kegel exercises and breathing methods. She also shared some of these exercises with her spouse, who was ready to help her during labor.

Due to "Expecting in Shape," Mamali felt inspired to take responsibility for her health throughout pregnancy. She was thankful for the information she acquired and felt confident in her ability to continue exercising safely after her kid was born.

The opening of "Expecting in Shape" establishes the book's tone and defines its goal. It starts by emphasizing the benefits of fitness during pregnancy and how it may help both the mother and the baby.

The introduction also addresses many women's worries and doubts about exercising during pregnancy, such as safety and what sorts of workouts are suited. It guarantees readers that the book will offer them the essential knowledge and guidance to exercise safely and confidently throughout pregnancy.

Furthermore, the introduction briefly outlines the book's different sections, such as understanding the changes in your body during pregnancy, safe exercise guidelines, designing an exercise program for pregnancy, nutrition and hydration during pregnancy, and preparing for labor and delivery through exercise.

The introduction finishes with a word of encouragement for pregnant women or hoping to become pregnant, underlining that exercising during pregnancy is safe and helpful for both the mother and the baby's health. Overall, the introduction sets the setting for an educational and practical guide for pregnant moms who desire to maintain their fitness levels throughout pregnancy.

1.1 Outline of the book

The "Expecting in Shape" summary offers readers a complete sense of what the book covers and how it might assist pregnant moms. The book emphasizes the value of exercising during pregnancy and how it may boost overall health and well-being for both the mother and the baby.

The book is structured into numerous parts, each addressing a distinct element of exercising during pregnancy. For example, readers will learn about the changes in the body during pregnancy, safe exercise standards, and building an exercise program ideal for their unique requirements.

The book also highlights the significance of good nutrition and hydration during pregnancy and includes practical suggestions on eating appropriately and remaining hydrated while exercising. Also, the book contains tips on managing typical pregnancy discomforts such as nausea, exhaustion, back pain, and leg cramps.

Additionally, the book tackles how exercising throughout pregnancy may prepare the body for labor and delivery and assist in postpartum recovery. It contains exercises that may help strengthen the pelvic floor muscles, strategies to aid with relaxation, and breathing exercises.

Overall, the summary of the book promotes "Expecting in Shape" as a thorough guide to fitness and well-being throughout pregnancy. It underscores the book's emphasis on giving pregnant moms practical guidance and safe workout instructions to encourage them to maintain a healthy lifestyle throughout pregnancy.

1.2 Importance of fitness during pregnancy

Pregnancy fitness is vital for the mother and the baby's well-being. Frequent physical exercise during pregnancy may improve cardiovascular function, lower the risk of gestational diabetes, and support healthy weight gain.

Additionally, keeping fit throughout pregnancy might help minimize the risk of pregnancy-related problems such as pre-eclampsia, gestational hypertension, and premature delivery. It may also help ease typical pregnant discomforts such as back pain, tiredness, and constipation.

Exercising during pregnancy might also bring emotional advantages. It may help decrease stress, anxiety, and sadness and enhance general mood and mental health. It also improves self-confidence and creates a feeling of empowerment and control over one's body during numerous changes.

Additionally, exercising throughout pregnancy might assist in preparing the body for labor and delivery. It may strengthen the pelvic floor muscles, enhance endurance, and promote flexibility, which can benefit an easier labor and delivery process.

Ultimately, the value of fitness throughout pregnancy cannot be emphasized. Frequent physical exercise may enhance both the mother's and the baby's health and give various physical and mental advantages. It is crucial for pregnant moms to obtain counsel from their healthcare professionals and to follow safe exercise recommendations while participating in physical activity during pregnancy.

Chapter Two

2.0 Benefits of Exercising During Pregnancy

2.1 Improving maternal health

Exercising during pregnancy can significantly improve maternal health. Regular physical activity can help reduce the risk of gestational diabetes, hypertension, and pre-eclampsia, common pregnancy-related complications. These conditions can be dangerous for the mother and the baby, so reducing their risk is crucial.

In addition, exercising during pregnancy can help maintain a healthy weight gain, which is vital for the mother's overall health and well-being. Excessive weight gain during pregnancy can increase the risk of complications such as gestational diabetes, hypertension, and pre-eclampsia.

Furthermore, regular exercise during pregnancy can help improve cardiovascular function, leading to increased blood flow and oxygenation for both the mother and the baby. It can also help improve insulin sensitivity, which can help prevent gestational diabetes.

Exercising during pregnancy can also help reduce the risk of postpartum depression. It can provide a sense of accomplishment and self-confidence and increase endorphins, the body's feel-good chemicals. Additionally, exercise may help improve sleep quality and decrease stress and anxiety, significant causes of postpartum depression.

Additionally, exercising throughout pregnancy might enhance the mother's general physical performance and mobility. Exercise may help preserve muscular strength and endurance, improve balance and coordination, and minimize the chance of falls, severe danger to pregnant women.

Lastly, consistent activity throughout pregnancy might assist in preparing the body for labor and delivery. It may help strengthen the pelvic floor muscles, which are vital for sustaining the baby's weight throughout pregnancy and during birth. It also boosts endurance and improves flexibility, benefiting the delivery procedure.

Overall, enhanced mother health is a considerable advantage of exercising during pregnancy. It may help avoid pregnancy-related problems, maintain a healthy weight gain, improve cardiovascular function, lower the risk of postpartum depression, increase physical function and mobility, and assist in labor and delivery.

2.2 Improved fetal health

Exercising throughout pregnancy may contribute to excellent fetal health. Frequent physical exercise may aid in enhancing blood flow and oxygenation to the baby, resulting in better fetal growth and development. It may also help minimize the risk of gestational diabetes, which can impact fetal development and raise the risk of difficulties during pregnancy and delivery.

Additionally, exercising throughout pregnancy might assist in boosting embryonic brain development. Research has indicated that regular pregnancy exercise may boost babies' cognitive performance and brain development.

Also, frequent activity throughout pregnancy might help minimize the chance of premature delivery. Preterm delivery is a substantial risk factor for infant death and morbidity, hence minimizing its risk is vital.

Exercising during pregnancy may also help minimize the chance of having a kid with a high birth weight. Infants born with a high birth weight are at a higher risk of childhood obesity and other health issues later in life.

Moreover, exercising during pregnancy may enhance the mother's general health and well-being, which can indirectly benefit fetal health. When the mother is healthy and well, she is better equipped to cater to the baby's requirements throughout pregnancy and after delivery.

Finally, exercising during pregnancy can help reduce the risk of complications during delivery. It can improve the mother's physical function and mobility, making it easier for her to deliver the baby. It can also help strengthen the pelvic floor muscles, reducing the risk of perineal tears and other birth injuries.

Generally, higher fetal health is a crucial advantage of exercising throughout pregnancy. It may increase fetal growth and development, lower the risk of preterm delivery and high birth weight, and contribute to better cognitive performance and brain Development in fetuses.

2.3 Easier labor and delivery

Exercising throughout pregnancy might make labor and delivery simpler for the mother. Frequent physical exercise may enhance cardiovascular function, muscular endurance, and flexibility, which are crucial for a healthy delivery.

Exercising during pregnancy may help strengthen the pelvic floor muscles necessary for sustaining the baby's weight throughout pregnancy and during the birth process. Strong pelvic floor muscles may help the woman push more efficiently during labor, lowering the risk of perineal tears and other birth complications.

Also, regular exercise throughout pregnancy helps boost endurance, which can assist the mother in remaining motivated during the long hours of labor. It may also enhance muscle control and coordination, which can assist the mother in maintaining appropriate posture and position throughout delivery. In addition, frequent exercise throughout pregnancy may help minimize the risk of interventions during labor and delivery, such as labor induction, instrumental delivery, and cesarean section. These procedures may raise the risk of problems and extend recovery time; thus, decreasing their requirement is suitable for both the mother and the infant.

Additionally, exercising during pregnancy may help decrease tension and anxiety, which can favor the delivery process. High stress and anxiety levels may interfere with labor and delivery; thus, minimizing their influence can simplify the process for the mother.

Lastly, frequent exercise throughout pregnancy may enhance the mother's general physical function and mobility, making it more straightforward for her to move about and change positions during labor and delivery.

Overall, smoother labor and delivery is a significant advantage of exercising throughout pregnancy. It may help strengthen the pelvic floor muscles, enhance endurance, minimize the need for interventions, reduce tension and anxiety, and improve general physical function and mobility.

2.4 Quicker postpartum recovery

Exercising during pregnancy may contribute to speedier postpartum recovery for the mother. Frequent physical exercise throughout pregnancy may improve general physical performance and preserve muscular strength, aiding recovery following delivery.

Following delivery, the body goes through a significant recuperation phase. Frequent exercise throughout pregnancy may assist in preparing the body for this healing process, making it more straightforward for the mother to return to her pre-pregnancy condition.

Frequent exercise throughout pregnancy may help strengthen the abdominal and pelvic floor muscles, commonly weakened during pregnancy and delivery. Stronger abdominal muscles may help the mother restore her pre-pregnancy abdominal tone more quickly. In comparison, stronger pelvic floor muscles can help lower the likelihood of urine incontinence and other pelvic floor issues.

Additionally, regular exercise throughout pregnancy may assist in enhancing cardiovascular function, which can aid in recovery after delivery. The improved blood flow and oxygenation may help decrease edema and inflammation and to improve recovery.

Additionally, regular exercise throughout pregnancy might help decrease stress and anxiety, which can positively influence postpartum recovery. High levels of stress and worry may interfere with healing; reducing their influence can make the process easier for the mother.

In addition, regular exercise throughout pregnancy might assist in increasing sleep quality and length, which is vital for a speedier postpartum recovery. Restful sleep is essential for healing and rebuilding energy levels.

Lastly, regular exercise throughout pregnancy may improve general physical function and mobility, making it more straightforward for the mother to care for her infant and accomplish everyday duties.

Overall, speedier postpartum recovery is a substantial advantage of exercising throughout pregnancy. It may help strengthen the abdomen and pelvic floor muscles, enhance cardiovascular function, decrease stress and anxiety, increase sleep quality, and improve general physical function and mobility.

Chapter Three

3.0 Understanding the Changes in Your Body During Pregnancy

Once upon a time, a young lady called Sarah was expecting her first child. As enthusiastic as she was about becoming a mother, she also felt a little overwhelmed by all the changes occurring in her body during pregnancy.

One day, Sarah was wandering through a bookshop when she came across a book titled "Understanding the Changes in Your Body during Pregnancy." Curious, she grabbed it up and began reading.

The book was full of excellent information regarding the changes throughout pregnancy, from hormonal swings to physical changes in the body. Sarah was shocked at how much she didn't know and how much there was to learn.

As she read on, Sarah knew that knowing these changes was vital for her to have a safe and happy pregnancy. She learned about the significance of prenatal care, proper eating choices, and frequent exercise. The book also outlined the many tests and procedures that will be done throughout pregnancy and why they are vital.

This newfound information made Sarah feel more secure and prepared for the voyage. She was able to negotiate the ups and downs of pregnancy more easily and appreciated the experience.

After her baby was born, Sarah was thankful for the book that had helped her comprehend the changes in her body throughout pregnancy. She suggested it to her friends and relatives who were expecting, knowing that it would be a helpful resource for anybody going through the same situation.

In the end, Sarah's golden experience with "Understanding the Changes in Your Body During Pregnancy" not only helped her have a healthy pregnancy but also gave her a newfound appreciation for the incredible changes her body underwent to bring her baby into the world.

3.1 Weight gain

Weight gain is a natural and necessary part of pregnancy. As the baby grows, the mother's body also undergoes significant changes to support the baby's development. However, excessive weight gain during pregnancy can increase the risk of complications, such as gestational diabetes, high blood pressure, and preterm birth.

The weight a woman should gain during pregnancy depends on her pre-pregnancy body mass index (BMI) (BMI). Women with a BMI in the normal range (18.5-24.9) should gain 25-35 pounds during pregnancy. Underweight women (BMI less than 18.5) should gain between 28-40 pounds, while women who are overweight (BMI between 25-29.9) should gain between 15-25 pounds. Women who are obese (BMI over 30) should aim for a weight gain of 11-20 pounds.

It is crucial to realize that weight increase during pregnancy is not simply attributable to the developing baby. Other factors, such as increased blood volume, amniotic fluid, and breast tissue, also contribute to weight gain. Additionally, women may experience increased appetite and cravings during pregnancy, leading to excess weight gain if not appropriately managed.

Maintaining a healthy and balanced diet is essential to manage weight gain during pregnancy. This involves ingesting various fruits, vegetables, lean portions of meat, entire grains, and healthy fats. It is also crucial to prevent excessive calorie consumption and restrict meals heavy in sugar and saturated fats.

Regular exercise during pregnancy can also help manage weight gain. Low-impact activities such as walking, swimming, and prenatal yoga can help maintain muscle tone and improve cardiovascular health. However, consulting with a healthcare provider before starting any exercise program during pregnancy is essential.

In conclusion, weight gain during pregnancy is a natural and necessary process. However, excessive weight gain can increase the risk of complications. By maintaining a healthy and balanced diet, managing cravings, and engaging in regular exercise, women can manage weight gain during pregnancy and promote a beneficial outcome for themselves and their babies.

3.2 Hormonal changes

Hormonal changes are a significant aspect of pregnancy, as the body goes through various shifts to support the baby's development. These hormonal changes start soon after conception and continue throughout pregnancy.

One of the primary hormones in pregnancy is human chorionic gonadotropin (hCG). This hormone is produced by the cells that form the placenta and is responsible for maintaining the pregnancy. It also plays a role in developing the baby's organs and stimulates the production of other hormones, such as estrogen and progesterone.

Estrogen is another hormone that plays a critical function in pregnancy. It helps to thicken the uterus lining, enhance blood flow to the uterus and placenta, and accelerate the formation of breast tissue.

Estrogen levels grow during pregnancy, reaching their most excellent value in the third trimester. Progesterone is also a crucial hormone during pregnancy. It helps to preserve the uterus lining and avoid contractions, which might lead to premature labor. Progesterone levels grow during pregnancy, peaking in the third trimester.

The rise in hormones during pregnancy may induce numerous physical and mental changes. For example, many women suffer morning sickness, which is assumed to be owing to the rise in hCG levels. Some frequent symptoms of hormonal changes during pregnancy include exhaustion, breast soreness, mood swings, and increased hunger.

Hormone changes during pregnancy might also impact the mother's mental health. Some women may have human chorionic gonadotropin (hCG) experience sadness or anxiety during pregnancy, which may be linked to hormonal fluctuations and the stress and changes connected with pregnancy.

In conclusion, hormonal changes are a vital element of pregnancy. They play a crucial role in the development of the infant and the physical and emotional changes experienced by the mother. Knowing these changes might help women prepare for the rigors of pregnancy and seek appropriate treatment when required.

3.2.1 Human chorionic gonadotropin (hCG)

Human chorionic gonadotropin (hCG) is a hormone generated by the cells that form the placenta during pregnancy. Its principal role is to sustain the pregnancy by promoting the synthesis of other hormones, such as estrogen and progesterone.

HCG levels may be identified in a woman's urine or blood as early as ten days after conception, making it a valuable marker for pregnancy testing. The stories of HCG in a woman's body rise fast during the first few weeks of pregnancy, doubling every 48 to 72 hours.

HCG is crucial in developing the baby's organs, notably the placenta. It helps to encourage the development of the placenta, which supplies the infant with the necessary nutrients and oxygen. HCG also governs the synthesis of other hormones essential for a healthy pregnancy.

Nevertheless, high levels of HCG may also suggest possible difficulties, such as molar or ectopic pregnancy. With a molar pregnancy, the placenta develops improperly, and there is no viable baby. In an ectopic pregnancy, the fertilized egg implants outside the uterus, which may be life-threatening if not treated swiftly.

In addition to its function in pregnancy, HCG has also been utilized for medical reasons, including treating infertility in men and women and as a marker for some forms of cancer, such as testicular and ovarian cancer.

In conclusion, HCG is a critical hormone in pregnancy, essential for sustaining the pregnancy and promoting the growth and development of the baby. Its levels may give vital information about the health of the pregnancy, and any variations from normal levels may demand additional research.

3.2.2 Estrogen

Estrogen is a hormone that is mainly generated by the ovaries but also by the placenta during pregnancy. It plays a vital role in developing and maintaining female sexual traits and reproductive function.

Estrogen levels grow considerably throughout pregnancy, reaching their peak in the third trimester. Estrogen helps to thicken the uterus lining, boost blood flow to the uterus and placenta, and encourage the formation of breast tissue. These modifications serve to promote the growth and development of the baby.

Estrogen also has a function in regulating other hormones, such as progesterone. It may help to inhibit ovulation during pregnancy, decreasing the production of future eggs and minimizing the likelihood of multiple pregnancies. Estrogen levels may also alter mood and behavior, resulting in changes in the mother's emotional state throughout pregnancy.

Yet, excessive amounts of estrogen during pregnancy might also pose significant hazards. High estrogen levels may contribute to gestational diabetes, pre-eclampsia, and early childbirth. Physicians and healthcare professionals must monitor estrogen levels throughout pregnancy and change therapy if required to avoid any unwanted effects.

Outside of pregnancy, estrogen also has a crucial impact on the menstrual cycle, bone density, and cholesterol levels. Decreased estrogen levels may contribute to menopausal symptoms, such as hot flashes, vaginal dryness, and bone loss. Hormone replacement therapy (HRT) can supplement estrogen levels in menopausal women, improving symptoms and reducing the risk of osteoporosis.

In conclusion, estrogen is a vital hormone during pregnancy, necessary for the growth and development of the baby and the mother's physical and emotional health. It also serves a key role in regulating reproductive function and sustaining general health in women. Understanding the effects of estrogen and monitoring levels during pregnancy and menopause is essential for optimal health and well-being.

3.2.3 Progesterone

Progesterone is a hormone that is primarily produced by the ovaries but also by the placenta during pregnancy. It is critical in sustaining a pregnancy and preparing the body for birthing.

Throughout pregnancy, progesterone levels grow considerably, reaching their peak in the third trimester. Progesterone helps to thicken the lining of the uterus, making it more receptive to implantation and aiding the formation of the placenta. It also helps to relax the muscles in the uterus, decreasing contractions and minimizing the risk of preterm labor.

Progesterone also controls the immune system and prevents the mother's body from rejecting the growing baby. It helps to suppress the mother's immune system to prevent it from attacking the fetus as a foreign organism.

Yet, low levels of progesterone during pregnancy might potentially have significant hazards. Insufficient progesterone levels may lead to miscarriage, premature labor, and other issues. Physicians and healthcare professionals must monitor progesterone levels throughout pregnancy and change therapy if required to avoid unwanted effects.

Outside of pregnancy, progesterone also plays a crucial part in the menstrual cycle and in preparing the body for pregnancy. It helps control the menstrual cycle, prepare the uterus for implantation, and stimulate breast tissue formation.

Progesterone is also used in hormone replacement treatment (HRT) to augment progesterone levels in menopausal women who have undergone a hysterectomy. Progesterone is required for women who take estrogen treatment since it helps to reduce the risk of uterine cancer.

In conclusion, progesterone is an essential hormone during pregnancy, necessary for the growth and development of the baby and the mother's physical and mental well-being. It also serves a key role in regulating reproductive function and sustaining general health in women. Understanding the effects of progesterone and monitoring levels during pregnancy and menopause is essential for optimal health and well-being.

3.3 Musculoskeletal changes

During pregnancy, the musculoskeletal system changes to support the growing fetus and prepare the mother's body for childbirth. Some of the significant changes that occur include:

The ovaries and the placenta produce relaxin hormones during pregnancy. It helps to relax the joints and ligaments in the pelvis and other body parts, allowing for greater flexibility and movement. However, this increased flexibility can also lead to joint instability and pain.

Center of gravity shift: As the baby grows, the mother's center of gravity shifts forward, increasing stress on the lower back and hips. This can lead to lower back pain and pelvic pain.

Abdominal muscle separation: The rectus abdominis muscles, commonly known as the "six-pack muscles," may separate during pregnancy to make room for the growing uterus. This separation, known as diastasis recti, can cause abdominal weakness and back pain.

Posture changes: The weight of the developing fetus may induce changes in posture, resulting in a more prominent curvature in the lower back, rounded shoulders, and a forward head position. These alterations may cause discomfort and pain in the neck, shoulders, and back.

Swelling and edema: During pregnancy, the body retains extra fluid, resulting in swelling and edema in the legs, feet, and hands. This may cause discomfort, agony, and problems with movement.

Increased risk of injury: Owing to the changes in the musculoskeletal system during pregnancy, there is an increased risk of injury, particularly in the lower back, hips, and knees. Taking adequate measures and seeking medical assistance is crucial to avoid or managing harm.

In conclusion, knowing the musculoskeletal changes during pregnancy is critical for managing pain and avoiding damage. Participating in proper exercise and physical therapy, keeping excellent posture, and getting medical assistance when required promote the mother's and infant's health and well-being.

Relaxin is a hormone generated by the ovaries and the placenta during pregnancy. Its primary role is to assist in relaxing the joints and ligaments in the pelvis and other regions of the body, allowing for increased flexibility and mobility. This increased flexibility is vital during labor, as it helps to accommodate the baby's journey down the birth canal.

In addition to its role in pregnancy, relaxin also plays a role in the menstrual cycle, ovulation, and other reproductive functions. It also has effects on other tissues and organs in the body, including the cardiovascular system, the respiratory system, and the immune system.

Throughout pregnancy, the levels of relaxin rise, peaking in the first trimester and continuing to increase throughout pregnancy. This increased production of relaxin may contribute to joint instability and discomfort, especially in the lower back, hips, and knees. It may also produce additional symptoms, such as greater flexibility in the feet and ankles, leading to foot discomfort and injury.

Although relaxin is crucial for promoting a healthy pregnancy and delivery, it may also harm the body. For example, increased relaxin production may contribute to joint instability and discomfort, making it difficult for pregnant women to remain active and healthy.

To control the effects of relaxin during pregnancy, it is crucial to participate in adequate exercise and physical therapy, maintain good posture, and seek medical assistance if required. By doing so, pregnant women may limit the pain and guarantee the health and well-being of both themselves and their newborns.

3.3.2 Center of gravity shift:

A woman's body experiences various changes during pregnancy, including a shift in her center of gravity. This shift happens when the baby develops and the uterus swells, exerting pressure on the pelvis and causing the abdomen to thrust forward. Consequently, a woman's weight distribution alters, and her center of gravity pushes forward.

This change might impact a woman's balance and coordination, making her more prone to falls and mishaps. It may also place extra tension on the back and pelvis muscles, producing pain and discomfort.
In addition, it may impair a woman's posture, resulting in a rounded back and shoulders and an increased risk of back discomfort.

Women need to participate in activities that strengthen the back, pelvis, and leg muscles to reduce the consequences of the center of gravity shift during pregnancy. This helps improve posture, minimize the risk of falls and accidents, and relieve pain and suffering.

It is also vital for pregnant women to be attentive to their movements and to take particular care while undertaking tasks that involve balance and coordination, such as climbing stairs or lifting heavy things. Choosing comfortable, supportive shoes and avoiding high heels may also enhance balance and minimize the chance of falls.

By being aware of the center of gravity shift and taking precautions to minimize its effects, pregnant women may remain active and healthy during their pregnancy and guarantee the well-being of themselves and their babies.

3.3.3 Abdominal muscle separation

Abdominal muscle separation, often known as diastasis recti, is a common problem during pregnancy. It is produced by the straining and weakening the connective tissue between the abdominal muscles as the uterus grows to accommodate the developing baby.

The separation may be aggravated by specific activities, such as heavy lifting or strenuous abdominal workouts, as well as by poor posture and alignment. In certain circumstances, it may also be attributed to hereditary factors or past abdominal surgery.

Abdominal muscle separation may produce various symptoms, including a bulging or projecting belly, lower back discomfort, and bad posture. It may also make it difficult to do some tasks, such as bending over or carrying heavy things.

To prevent or manage abdominal muscle separation during pregnancy, it is necessary to participate in adequate exercise and physical therapy, maintain good posture, and avoid activities that place undue tension on the abdominal muscles. This may entail skipping workouts such as crunches and sit-ups and concentrating on exercises that strengthen the pelvic floor and other core muscles.

Surgery may be required to reconnect the split abdominal muscles in extreme situations. Yet, in most cases, the illness may be controlled with non-invasive means, such as exercise and physical therapy.

It is crucial for pregnant women to be aware of the signs of abdominal muscle separation and to seek medical assistance if required. By doing so, women may limit the pain and guarantee the health and well-being of themselves and their kids.

Posture changes are typical during pregnancy and may be caused by some causes, including weight increase, hormone changes, and musculoskeletal abnormalities. As the baby develops and the uterus swells, the center of gravity slips forward, leading to a change in posture to maintain balance.

Pregnant women may suffer an increase in the curvature of the lower back, contributing to lower back discomfort. The chest may grow more rounded, and the shoulders may slide forward. These posture variations may disrupt the spine's alignment and raise the risk of back pain and other musculoskeletal disorders.

Women must follow healthy posture practices to limit the risk of posture-related pain during pregnancy. This may involve standing up straight with the shoulders back and down, activating the core muscles to support the spine, and avoiding slouching or leaning forward excessively.

Physical therapy and exercise may also help improve posture during pregnancy. Stretching and strengthening activities increase flexibility and muscular strength, supporting the spine and maintaining a healthy posture.

In rare circumstances, specialist equipment, like a pregnancy support belt, may be prescribed to give extra support for the developing belly and reduce strain on the lower back.

By adopting good posture practices and getting appropriate medical treatment, pregnant women may limit the risk of pain and musculoskeletal disorders associated with posture changes during pregnancy.

3.3.5 Swelling and edema:

Swelling and edema are frequent during pregnancy and may be caused by several causes, including hormonal changes and increased strain on the veins and lymphatic system.

The body generates extra blood and bodily fluids during pregnancy to support the developing baby, possibly contributing to edema and fluid retention. Hormone shifts may also alter the body's capacity to control fluid levels, resulting in further edema.

Swelling is most frequent in the feet, ankles, and legs but may also occur in other body regions, such as the hands and face. In rare circumstances, swelling may be substantial and contribute to pain and movement concerns.

To limit the risk of swelling and edema during pregnancy, it is vital to keep active and prevent long periods of sitting or standing. Elevating the feet and receiving frequent activity, such as walking or swimming, may assist in improving circulation and prevent fluid accumulation.

Choosing comfortable, supportive footwear and avoiding tight clothes may also lower the risk of edema. In certain circumstances, compression stockings may be prescribed to aid in improving circulation and minimize the risk of edema.

In most situations, swelling and edema are not the reason for worry and may be treated with easy lifestyle adjustments. Nevertheless, suppose swelling is significant or accompanied by other symptoms, such as high blood pressure or headaches. In that case, it is crucial to seek medical assistance to rule out any underlying health concerns.

3.3.6 Greater Chance of Harm

Throughout pregnancy, the body experiences various changes that might raise the risk of damage. Hormone changes may increase flexibility and joint laxity, making strain or spraining muscles and ligaments easier. Moreover, the additional weight and altered center of gravity may compromise balance and coordination, increasing the risk of falls and other mishaps.

To limit the risk of injury during pregnancy, it is necessary to participate in regular activity and maintain excellent posture. Strengthening activities may aid in supporting the joints and muscles, while balance and coordination exercises can enhance general stability.

It is also vital to take additional care while participating in physical activities, such as avoiding high-impact workouts or exercises that demand quick changes in direction or movement. Using adequate footwear and protective gear may also assist in limiting the chance of injury.

If an accident does occur, it is crucial to seek medical assistance swiftly to avoid additional consequences. In certain circumstances, adjustments to exercise regimens or physical treatment may be essential to assist recovery and prevent future damage.

Overall, remaining aware of the increased risk of injury during pregnancy and adopting proper measures will assist in ensuring a safe and healthy pregnancy. By being active, maintaining good posture, and avoiding injury, pregnant moms may decrease the risk of difficulties and have a happy, healthy pregnancy.

Chapter Four

4.0 Safe Exercise Recommendations During Pregnancy

4.1 Varieties of workouts suggested during pregnancy

Keeping active throughout pregnancy may assist in boosting overall health and wellness for the mother and the growing baby. Nevertheless, not all workouts are suitable for expecting moms, and it is crucial to contact a healthcare expert before starting any new exercise plan.

Some forms of workouts that are typically safe and advised during pregnancy include:

Walking: This low-impact activity is a fantastic way to keep active throughout pregnancy. It can assist in enhancing cardiovascular health, maintaining muscular tone, and boosting overall endurance.

Swimming: Swimming and water aerobics may be a terrific way to keep active while decreasing the chance of injury or strain. The buoyancy of the water may aid in supporting the body and alleviate stress on the joints.

Prenatal yoga may increase flexibility, strength, and balance while encouraging relaxation and stress reduction. Prenatal yoga programs are customized particularly to the requirements of pregnant moms, with modified postures and breathing practices meant to assist pregnancy and delivery.

Strength training: Mild strength training activities might assist in maintaining muscle tone and support the joints during pregnancy. Exercises focusing on the core, hips, and back may be efficient.

Low-impact aerobics: Low-impact aerobics, such as stationary cycling or elliptical training, may enhance cardiovascular health and maintain general fitness throughout pregnancy.

It is vital to avoid high-impact or contact sports and workouts that demand quick changes in direction or movement. Moreover, activities that entail resting flat on the back or standing for lengthy periods should be avoided after the first trimester.

Overall, being active and involved in regular exercise throughout pregnancy may assist in maintaining general health and wellness for both the mother and baby. By speaking with a healthcare physician and participating in safe, suitable exercise regimens, expecting moms may experience a pleasant and healthy pregnancy.

4.1.1 Walking

Walking is a low-impact activity usually considered safe and recommended for pregnant women. It may promote cardiovascular health, maintain muscular tone, and boost overall endurance.

Walking during pregnancy may also assist in relieving stress and anxiety, support healthy weight growth, and prepare the body for birth and delivery. It is crucial to wear comfortable, supportive shoes and clothes while walking and to avoid walking on uneven or slippery terrain.

Expectant moms should strive to walk for at least 30 minutes a day, preferably at a moderate pace. If required, this may be split up into shorter periods, such as three 10-minute walks throughout the day.

Yet, pregnant women must listen to their bodies and adapt their walking regimen as required. Women who encounter difficulties during pregnancy, such as premature labor, should check with their healthcare professional before participating in any fitness regimen, including walking.

Walking is a safe and effective strategy for pregnant women to keep active and boost overall health and wellness. Expectant moms may experience a pleasant and healthy pregnancy by including frequent walking into their routine.

4.1.2 Swimming

Swimming is another low-impact activity that is highly suggested for pregnant women. It is a terrific approach to enhancing cardiovascular endurance and general muscular strength while reducing stress on the joints and ligaments.

Swimming during pregnancy may also assist in easing typical pregnancy-related symptoms such as back discomfort, edema, and exhaustion. Finding a comfortable swimsuit that offers appropriate support for the developing tummy is crucial.

Expectant moms should strive to swim for at least 30 minutes a day, three to five days a week. Swimming in a pool that is heated to a suitable temperature is advisable since the body temperature during pregnancy is more significant than usual.

Pregnant women should also be careful while swimming and avoid diving or leaping into the pool, as well as other activities that entail rapid changes in direction or effort. Avoid swimming in overly hot water, such as a hot tub or sauna, is also vital.

Like any fitness regimen during pregnancy, it is vital to contact a healthcare physician before commencing a swimming routine, especially if there are any underlying health problems or difficulties.
Swimming is a safe and effective approach for pregnant women to keep active and boost overall health and wellness. Expectant moms may experience a pleasant and healthy pregnancy by including frequent swimming into their regimen.

4.1.3 Prenatal yoga

Prenatal yoga is a mild exercise that is mainly developed for pregnant women. It is a terrific approach to induce relaxation, decrease stress, and increase flexibility and strength during pregnancy.
Prenatal yoga sessions often contain a sequence of mild stretches, postures, and breathing exercises that are safe and useful for pregnant women. Several yoga postures may be altered to suit a developing belly and other physical changes associated with pregnancy.

In addition to its physical advantages, prenatal yoga may also assist in preparing pregnant moms for childbirth by fostering calm and deep breathing methods that can be employed throughout labor and delivery. It may also help to ease typical pregnancy-related symptoms such as back discomfort, nausea, and exhaustion.

Pregnant women must pick a skilled and experienced prenatal yoga teacher who can assist them through a safe and productive practice. Women should also advise their teacher about any underlying health concerns or difficulties that may necessitate changes or adjustments to their yoga practice.

Expectant moms may practice prenatal yoga throughout their pregnancy, with adjustments as required. Practicing prenatal yoga at least two to three times weekly is suggested for the best effects.

Overall, prenatal yoga is a safe and beneficial approach for pregnant women to keep active, decrease stress, and prepare for delivery. By including regular prenatal yoga, expectant moms may experience a more pleasant and healthier pregnancy.

4.1.4 Strength training

Strength training, often known as resistance training, is a kind of exercise that includes utilizing weights or resistance to increase muscular strength and endurance. It is a safe and efficient technique for pregnant women to maintain their fitness and prepare for delivery.

Throughout pregnancy, women suffer changes in their body composition, including increased body weight and a shift in the center of gravity. Strength exercise may assist in maintaining muscle mass and improve balance and stability, lowering the risk of falls and injury.

Strength training activities may include weight lifting, bodyweight workouts, and resistance bands. Expectant moms should concentrate on low-impact exercises that avoid exerting undue stress on their joints or abdominal muscles.

Pregnant women should contact their healthcare professionals before commencing any strength training program. It is crucial to start with small weights and progressively increase the intensity and volume of the workouts. Women should also avoid holding their breath during strength training and should take pauses as required to prevent overexertion.

Frequent strength exercise may assist in decreasing typical pregnancy-related symptoms such as back discomfort and exhaustion. It may help increase general fitness and prepare women for the physical rigors of birth and delivery.

Strength training is a safe and effective strategy for pregnant women to maintain their fitness and prepare for delivery. By incorporating regular strength training into their routine, expectant mothers can enjoy a more comfortable and healthy pregnancy.

4.1.5 Low-impact aerobics

Low-impact aerobics involves movements that do not require a lot of jumping or jarring motions, making it safe and effective training for pregnant women. This exercise can help maintain cardiovascular health, strengthen muscles, and improve flexibility.

During pregnancy, hormonal changes can cause the heart to work harder, and low-impact aerobics can help improve cardiovascular fitness without too much stress on the body. Additionally, low-impact aerobics can help to maintain a healthy weight, which is essential for both the mother and the baby.

Low-impact aerobics can include activities such as brisk walking, cycling, and swimming. These low-impact activities help maintain cardiovascular health without placing too much strain on the joints or abdominal muscles. Other low-impact aerobics activities include dancing, elliptical machines, and low-impact aerobics classes.

Expectant moms should contact their healthcare professionals before commencing any fitness regimen. Starting with low to moderate-intensity exercise is crucial, and progressively increasing the length and intensity over time is vital. Women should also listen to their bodies and relax to avoid overexertion.

Regular low-impact aerobics may assist in easing typical pregnancy-related problems such as back discomfort, constipation, and exhaustion. It may help increase general fitness and prepare women for the physical rigors of birth and delivery.

Overall, low-impact aerobics is a safe and effective strategy for pregnant women to maintain their fitness and prepare for delivery. Including regular low-impact aerobics, expectant moms may experience a more pleasant and healthier pregnancy.

4.2   Exercises to avoid during pregnancy

Although exercise during pregnancy is vital, particular kinds of workouts should be avoided since they may place too much stress on the body and damage the growing baby. These are several workouts to avoid during pregnancy:

Contact sports: Games such as soccer, basketball, and hockey, where there is a chance of getting struck in the abdomen, should be avoided.

High-impact exercises: Exercises like jumping jacks, high-intensity aerobics, and sprinting on hard surfaces might be too jarring on the joints and should be avoided.

Exercises that demand laying on your back: As your pregnancy continues, it is not advisable to undertake activities that need you to rest on your back for lengthy durations. This is because the developing fetus's weight may strain the vena cava, the central vein that transports blood back to the heart from the lower body, possibly decreasing blood supply to the infant.

Hot yoga or hot Pilates: Practicing in a hot and humid atmosphere may elevate your core body temperature, which can be hazardous to the fetus. It is advisable to avoid workouts in conditions exceeding 90 degrees Fahrenheit.

Scuba diving: Scuba diving may lead to decompression sickness, which can be dangerous to both the mother and the fetus.
It is crucial to discuss any fitness regimen with your healthcare professional to ensure that you are practicing workouts that are safe for both you and your developing baby.

4.2.1 Contact sports

Contact sports are often high-impact and include a lot of physical contact with opponents, such as football, soccer, basketball, and hockey. Certain sports are not advised during pregnancy because they raise the risk of damage to the mother and the growing baby.

Physical contact may occur in falls, strikes to the abdomen, and other trauma, which can cause significant injury to the baby. Moreover, contact sports demand a lot of twisting, turning, and rapid movements that may strain the joints and ligaments, increasing the risk of damage to the mother.

Pregnant women need to avoid contact sports and instead concentrate on low-impact and low-risk workouts, like walking, swimming, and prenatal yoga. These activities give various health advantages without excessive stress on the body or the growing baby. It is always vital for pregnant women to check with their healthcare professional before beginning any fitness program to verify that it is safe and suitable for their unique requirements and health condition.

High-impact workouts include activities that impose a large amount of stress on the joints and bones, such as running, leaping, and aerobics. These workouts are not suggested for pregnant women since they raise the risk of damage to both the mother and the growing baby. The impact may inflict stress on the joints and ligaments, resulting in injury or pain. Moreover, high-impact activities might raise the chance of falls, which can be especially hazardous during pregnancy.

Instead of high-impact workouts, pregnant women should concentrate on low-impact exercises that give numerous health advantages without placing excessive stress on the body or the growing baby. Walking, swimming, and prenatal yoga are all terrific alternatives for low-impact workouts. These exercises assist in preserving cardiovascular health, building muscular strength, and developing flexibility and balance.

Pregnant women need to review their exercise plans with their healthcare practitioner to ensure they are safe and suitable for their unique requirements and health conditions. Pregnant women engaging in high-impact activities should speak to their healthcare professional about altering their routine or switching to lower-impact exercises to limit the risk of damage to themselves and their growing baby.

During pregnancy, avoiding workouts that entail laying on your back for longer durations is crucial. This is because the weight of the uterus and baby might compress the vena cava, a large vein that transfers blood from the lower body to the heart. This may restrict the blood supply to the baby and can cause dizziness, shortness of breath, and nausea in the mother. Activities involving reclining on your back, like classic sit-ups or crunches, should be avoided after the first trimester.

Alternatively, pregnant women may choose modified workouts that can be conducted in a side-lying posture or in a reclined position with the upper body raised. These may include modified Pilates exercises, like pelvic tilts, sitting leg lifts, or pregnant yoga postures that can be practiced in a reclined or side-lying position. Contacting a healthcare physician before commencing any fitness regimen during pregnancy is crucial.

4.2.4 Hot Yoga or Hot Pilates

Hot yoga or hot Pilates, which entail practicing yoga or Pilates in a heated setting, are not suggested during pregnancy. The high temperature may elevate the mother's core body temperature and damage the growing fetus. In addition, the heat may induce dehydration and raise the risk of dizziness and fainting.

Pregnant women should also avoid hot tubs, saunas, and steam rooms, since these may significantly elevate the body temperature and contribute to dehydration. Maintaining a healthy body temperature and keeping well-hydrated throughout pregnancy is crucial to assist fetal growth and avoiding problems.

Alternatively, pregnant women may choose prenatal yoga or Pilates sessions that are particularly tailored for pregnancy and are taught by licensed teachers. These programs often feature gentle motions, breathing exercises, and relaxation methods that may help ease pain and stress during pregnancy.

4.2.5 Scuba diving

Scuba diving is a sport that requires diving underwater while inhaling via a scuba tank. This activity is not advised during pregnancy because of the danger of decompression sickness, popularly known as "the bends." Decompression sickness is caused by nitrogen bubbles developing in the blood and tissues owing to the sudden fall in pressure that happens during ascent after a dive.

During pregnancy, there is a higher risk of decompression sickness because the body's tissues absorb nitrogen more quickly, and the baby may be in danger of fetal hypoxia owing to the alterations in gas exchange that occur while diving. In addition, scuba diving entails physical activity and raises the chance of injury, which may be particularly harmful during pregnancy. Hence, pregnant women should avoid scuba diving and other high-risk activities that require fast pressure changes or physical effort.

4.3 Adjustments for various stages of pregnancy

Exercising during pregnancy may be incredibly helpful, but altering your routine as your body changes during each trimester is vital. These are some alterations to consider during each stage of pregnancy:

First Trimester:

Throughout the first trimester, it's vital to concentrate on low-impact workouts like walking, swimming, and prenatal yoga. Avoiding activities that entail resting on your back for long periods is also essential. While your body adapts to the changes, be careful to listen to your body and prevent overexertion.

Second Trimester:

As your baby bulge develops, you may need to change your regimen to fit your changing physique. Try adding pelvic floor exercises to your regimen to aid with bladder control and support your developing tummy. You may also need to alter activities that involve balance, such as lunges or squats, by holding onto a steady surface or utilizing a wider stance.

Third Trimester:

Throughout the third trimester, it's crucial to concentrate on workouts that prepare your body for labor and delivery. Add activities that strengthen your hips and pelvic floor muscles, like squats or Kegels. It's also vital to avoid workouts that exert too much pressure on your body, such as deep squats or leaping. Generally, it's crucial to listen to your body and alter your workout plan as required during each stage of pregnancy. Speak with your healthcare practitioner and a trained prenatal fitness specialist to establish a safe and effective workout regimen.

Chapter Five

5.0 Creating a Workout Program for Pregnancy

5.1 Establishing fitness objectives during Pregnancy

Establishing exercise goals throughout pregnancy is vital to maintaining a healthy lifestyle for both the mother and the developing baby. It is crucial to remember that fitness objectives during pregnancy should differ from those during pre-pregnancy or postpartum periods. The aims should be maintaining a healthy weight, enhancing stamina, improving flexibility, and lowering stress.

Contacting a healthcare expert before establishing any exercise objectives during pregnancy is essential since every woman's body is different and may need extraordinary changes. The provider may aid in detecting any possible hazards or restrictions and advise suitable workouts appropriately.

Some examples of fitness objectives during pregnancy include:

1. **Keeping a healthy weight:** Gaining weight is a regular aspect of pregnancy, but ensuring it is within safe limits is crucial. The healthcare professional might advise on the appropriate weight increase during pregnancy depending on the mother's pre-pregnancy BMI.

2. **Enhancing cardiovascular health:** Exercises such as brisk walking, swimming, or low-impact aerobics aid in improving cardiovascular health and building stamina.

3. **Strengthening muscles:** Strength training activities utilizing small weights or resistance bands may increase muscular strength and tone, particularly in the legs, back, and pelvic area.

4. **Increasing flexibility:** Prenatal yoga and stretching activities may aid in developing flexibility, decreasing muscular tension, and improving general posture.

5. **Lowering stress:** Participating in relaxing activities such as prenatal massage, meditation, or deep breathing exercises may aid in decreasing tension and generating a feeling of peace.

It is crucial to create reasonable and attainable exercise objectives throughout pregnancy and heed the body's suggestions. It is also essential to keep hydrated, wear appropriate clothes and shoes, and avoid exercising in harsh weather conditions or high altitudes.

5.1.1 Keeping a healthy weight

Keeping a healthy weight during pregnancy is vital for the health of both the mother and the baby. It is natural to gain weight during pregnancy, but excessive weight gain may lead to health concerns for both the mother and the baby.

The weight a woman should acquire during pregnancy depends on her pre-pregnancy weight and body mass index (BMI) (BMI). Underweight women should receive more weight than those who are overweight or obese. On average, women with a healthy pre-pregnancy weight should gain between 25 and 35 pounds during pregnancy.

Keeping a healthy weight may be done through good food and frequent exercise. Consuming a well-balanced diet that contains a range of fruits, vegetables, whole grains, lean meats, and healthy fats may offer the required nutrients for both the mother and the baby. It is vital to avoid foods that are rich in saturated and trans fats and meals that are high in sugar.

Exercise may also assist in maintaining a healthy weight during pregnancy. Moderate-intensity activities such as brisk walking, swimming, and yoga may help to burn calories and keep the body healthy. It is vital to check with a healthcare physician before starting or maintaining any fitness regimen during pregnancy since certain activities may not suit pregnant women.

It is also vital to avoid crash diets or severe weight loss during pregnancy since this may be hazardous to the baby's health. Instead, concentrate on making healthy choices and lifestyle improvements that can be maintained long-term. Frequent prenatal check-ups with a healthcare practitioner may assist in monitoring weight growth and safeguard the health of the mother and the baby.

5.1.2 Enhancing cardiovascular health

Optimizing cardiovascular health during pregnancy is vital for both the mother and the baby. Frequent physical exercise may help minimize the risk of heart disease, high blood pressure, and gestational diabetes. It also helps to enhance stamina and energy levels, which may be advantageous during labor and delivery.

Various workouts help promote cardiovascular health, such as walking, swimming, low-impact aerobics, and cycling. The American College of Obstetricians and Gynecologists suggests that pregnant women strive for at least 150 minutes of moderate-intensity weekly aerobic exercise. This may be reached with 30 minutes of activity on most days of the week.

It is vital to start softly and progressively increase the intensity and length of the exercise as the pregnancy advances. Women not physically active before pregnancy should check with their healthcare physician before commencing any fitness regimen. Women with specific medical issues or pregnancy difficulties may need to avoid certain forms of activity or adjust their exercise schedule.

It is also vital to remain hydrated during exercise and to avoid exercising in high temperatures. Women should listen to their bodies and stop exercising if they encounter discomfort, dizziness, or shortness of breath. Frequent exercise and a good diet may assist in improving cardiovascular health and general wellness throughout pregnancy.

5.1.3 Strengthening muscles

Strengthening muscles during pregnancy may assist in supporting the increased weight and changes in posture, minimize the chance of injury, and make it simpler to carry out everyday duties. Resistance training, such as dumbbells, resistance bands, or bodyweight exercises, may help build key muscular groups, including the legs, arms, back, and core.

Throughout pregnancy, it's crucial to concentrate on low-impact activities that prevent exerting undue pressure on the joints and ligaments. Bodyweight exercises like squats, lunges, and planks are terrific for building muscles without unnecessary stress. Resistance bands may also be used to increase resistance to motions like bicep curls or shoulder presses.

Engaging with a trained fitness expert or healthcare physician is crucial to building a strength training program that is safe and suitable for each trimester of pregnancy. As the body changes during pregnancy, adaptations may need to be made to workouts and the amount of weight employed. In addition, avoiding activities that entail resting flat on the back is vital since this might limit blood supply to the uterus and perhaps injure the baby.

5.1.4 Enhancing flexibility

Developing flexibility is an essential element of a well-rounded workout regimen during pregnancy. When the body experiences physical changes, muscles and joints may become tight and inflexible, leading to pain and even damage. Frequent stretching exercises help increase flexibility and avoid these difficulties.

Pregnancy-specific stretching exercises may target regions such as the lower back, hips, thighs, and shoulders, which are typically impacted by the physical changes that occur during pregnancy. Moderate stretching motions concentrating on the main muscle groups may help reduce stress and enhance circulation.

Some common stretches during pregnancy include hamstring stretches, hip flexor stretches, and spinal twists. It's vital to emphasize that times should be done softly and gradually, without bouncing or pushing the body into postures that produce pain or discomfort. Holding each stretch for 20-30 seconds and repeating it 2-3 times may help develop flexibility.

Prenatal yoga is also an extraordinary approach to increasing flexibility during pregnancy. Many yoga positions concentrate on stretching and extending muscles while fostering relaxation and stress alleviation. But, it's vital to find a prenatal yoga session that is mainly developed for pregnant women and guided by a competent teacher.

In addition to improving flexibility, regular stretching exercises may also assist in preparing the body for labor by increasing pelvic mobility and minimizing the chance of perineal tearing. Like any fitness regimen during pregnancy, it's vital to consult a healthcare expert before beginning and heed the body's requirements and restrictions.

5.1.5 Managing stress

Pregnancy may be a trying time for many women, both physically and psychologically. Exercise has been demonstrated to be an excellent technique for relieving stress during pregnancy. Regular physical activity helps lower levels of stress hormones such as cortisol and promotes the synthesis of endorphins, which are feel-good chemicals that can enhance mood.

In addition to exercising, additional ways might assist in alleviating stress during pregnancy. They include relaxation methods such as deep breathing, meditation, and visualization. It's also vital to take time for yourself and indulge in things you love, whether reading a book, taking a bath, or spending time with friends.

It's worth mentioning that although exercise may be a terrific method to alleviate stress during pregnancy, it's crucial not to overdo it. High-intensity exercise or pushing oneself too hard might raise stress levels and be counterproductive. It's critical to listen to your body and take pauses when required

5.2 Creating a Regimen that meets your requirements

Establishing a fitness regimen during pregnancy is vital to maintaining a healthy lifestyle for both the mother and the baby. While designing a workout regimen, it is crucial to consider the particular requirements of the mother and any constraints or advice from a healthcare practitioner.

One essential issue to examine is the mother's fitness level before pregnancy. People who were active before getting pregnant may be able to continue with a similar schedule with minor alterations. Nevertheless, it is necessary for people who were not active before pregnancy to start with low-impact workouts and gradually build intensity over time.

Another critical aspect is the stage of pregnancy. As the pregnancy proceeds, the body experiences changes that may influence exercise capacity and comfort level. For example, some workouts may become more brutal or painful when the belly grows. While developing a fitness program, it is crucial to integrate a range of exercises to target various muscle groups and maintain overall fitness. These may include aerobic workouts such as walking or swimming, strength training exercises with small weights or resistance bands, and stretching or yoga techniques for flexibility and relaxation.

It is also vital to listen to the body and make alterations as required. If an activity causes discomfort or agony, altering or removing that exercise from the regimen may be essential.
Ultimately, developing a fitness program during pregnancy is about striking a balance between keeping active and healthy and emphasizing the health and safety of both the mother and the baby.

5.3 Scheduling exercise sessions

Scheduling exercise sessions during pregnancy is vital to maintaining a regular exercise routine. It's recommended that pregnant women engage in moderate-intensity exercise for at least 150 minutes per week, which can be broken down into 30-minute sessions five days a week.

When scheduling exercise sessions, it's essential to consider your energy levels and other commitments throughout the day. Many women find it helpful to exercise in the morning when they have more energy before other daily tasks pile up. However, if you have morning sickness or are more energetic later in the day, you should schedule your exercise sessions accordingly.

Additionally, it's essential to make time for rest and recovery. Pregnancy can be tiring and demanding on the body, so it's necessary to listen to your body and take breaks when needed. This may mean scheduling rest days between exercise sessions or modifying the intensity and duration of your workouts.

Building a routine that suits your needs and schedule is critical to regular exercise during pregnancy. It's essential to prioritize your health and well-being while also considering any limitations or recommendations from your healthcare provider.

Chapter Six

6.0 Nutrition and Hydration During Pregnancy

6.1 The importance of a balanced diet during pregnancy

A balanced diet during pregnancy is essential for the health of both the mother and the growing fetus. Eating various nutrient-rich foods ensures the mother and the baby receive the necessary vitamins, minerals, and other nutrients for proper growth and development.

Protein is an essential food during pregnancy since it is necessary for developing and repairing tissues in both the mother and the fetus. Excellent sources of protein include lean meats, poultry, fish, eggs, beans, and legumes.

Calcium is vital for forming strong bones and teeth in the growing embryo. Dairy products, including milk, cheese, and yogurt, are good providers of calcium. Additional sources of calcium include leafy greens, tofu, fortified drinks, and cereals.

Iron is essential for the synthesis of red blood cells and the prevention of anemia during pregnancy. Iron-rich foods include lean meats, poultry, fish, beans, fortified cereals, and leafy greens. Vitamin C may aid with iron absorption; therefore, consuming foods high in vitamin C, including citrus fruits, tomatoes, and bell peppers, might be helpful.

Folic acid is vital for the early development of the neural tube and may help avoid birth abnormalities. Excellent sources of folic acid include leafy greens, fortified cereals, beans, and lentils.

In addition to these nutrients, consuming a variety of fruits, vegetables, whole grains, and healthy fats is crucial throughout pregnancy. Avoiding processed and sugary meals is also vital for a healthy pregnancy. It's also vital for pregnant women to keep hydrated by drinking lots of water throughout the day. Proper hydration may help avoid constipation, a frequent condition during pregnancy.

Overall, a balanced and nutrient-rich diet during pregnancy may assist in improving the health of both the mother and the baby. It's always preferable to check with a healthcare physician or trained dietitian for individualized dietary advice throughout pregnancy.

Protein is a macronutrient that plays a critical function in creating, repairing, and maintaining tissues in the body. It is made up of amino acids, which are the building blocks of protein. During pregnancy, protein is particularly critical for fetal growth and development and for maintaining the mother's increased blood volume and breast tissue.

Pregnant women are encouraged to eat an additional 25 grams of protein per day compared to non-pregnant women, corresponding to roughly 75-100 grams of protein per day. Excellent protein sources include lean meats, poultry, fish, eggs, dairy products, beans, legumes, nuts, and seeds.

It's crucial to know that specific protein sources may also contain high quantities of mercury or other pollutants, which may be detrimental to the growing baby. Pregnant women should avoid high-mercury fish such as shark, swordfish, king mackerel, and tilefish and restrict their diet of other fish and seafood to 2-3 servings per week.

Also, pregnant women should be careful about ingesting raw or undercooked meat, chicken, fish, and eggs since these may be sources of hazardous germs such as Salmonella and Listeria. It's also crucial to implement appropriate food hygiene and sanitation procedures to limit the risk of foodborne disease.

6.1.2 Calcium

Calcium is vital for forming strong bones and teeth, regulating heart function, and assisting muscle function. During pregnancy, calcium is crucial for the development of the baby's bones and teeth and the mother's health.

The recommended daily calcium intake during pregnancy is 1,000-1,300 milligrams (mg), depending on the mother's age and health state. Excellent dietary sources of calcium include dairy products such as milk, cheese, and yogurt, leafy green vegetables, tofu, almonds, and calcium-fortified foods such as orange juice and cereal.

If a pregnant woman is not able to receive enough calcium from her diet, calcium supplements may be advised by her healthcare professional. It's vital to consult a healthcare practitioner before taking any supplements during pregnancy to verify they are safe and effective.

6.1.3 Iron

Iron is a vital component that is critical in producing red blood cells and carrying oxygen throughout the body. During pregnancy, a woman's body needs an increased quantity of iron to support the growth and development of the baby and the expansion of the maternal blood supply.

Iron deficiency anemia is a prevalent illness among pregnant women, and it may lead to issues such as premature delivery, low birth weight, and postpartum depression. Thus, it is crucial for pregnant women to eat adequate iron-rich meals or take iron supplements as suggested by their healthcare professionals.

Some healthy sources of iron are lean red meat, chicken, fish, lentils, beans, tofu, spinach, and fortified breakfast cereals. Taking vitamin C-rich meals combined with iron-rich foods is also suggested to boost iron absorption.

Pregnant women should take at least 27 mg of iron daily. Nevertheless, some women may need more iron supplements if they risk developing iron deficiency anemia. It is vital to consult a healthcare expert to establish the optimum quantity of iron consumption during pregnancy.

Folic acid, often known as folate or vitamin B9, is vital for pregnant women. It is necessary for correct fetal brain and spine development, particularly during the first trimester of pregnancy. Folic acid is also essential for creating red blood cells and DNA synthesis.

Pregnant women must ingest 400-800 micrograms (mcg) of folic acid daily. This may be gained via a balanced diet that includes leafy green vegetables, beans, citrus fruits, and fortified cereals. Nevertheless, many women take a daily folic acid pill to guarantee appropriate consumption.

A shortage in folic acid during pregnancy may contribute to neural tube abnormalities, such as spina bifida, in the growing baby. It may also raise the risk of early delivery and poor birth weight. Consequently, pregnant women must prioritize receiving adequate folic acid in their diet or via supplements.

6.2 Foods to avoid during pregnancy

Throughout pregnancy, it is vital to avoid specific meals to maintain the growing baby's health. Some of the items to avoid include:

Raw or undercooked meat: Raw or undercooked meat may contain hazardous germs such as E. coli or Salmonella, which can cause food poisoning.

Deli meats and processed meat: These sorts of flesh may also contain hazardous germs and should be avoided unless roasted to an internal temperature of 165°F (74°C).

Fish with high amounts of mercury: Some varieties of fish, such as shark, swordfish, king mackerel, and tilefish, have high levels of mercury, which may impair the developing neural system of the newborn.

Raw or undercooked eggs: Raw or undercooked eggs may carry Salmonella, which can cause food poisoning.

Soft cheeses: Soft cheeses such as Brie, Camembert, and feta may contain Listeria, a bacterium that can cause miscarriage or stillbirth.

Unpasteurized dairy products: Unpasteurized dairy products might contain dangerous bacteria and should be avoided during pregnancy.

Raw sprouts: Raw sprouts like alfalfa, clover, and radish might contain hazardous germs such as E. coli or Salmonella.

Caffeine: Excessive amounts of caffeine consumption during pregnancy have been associated with low birth weight and miscarriage. It is suggested to restrict caffeine consumption to fewer than 200 mg per day.

Alcohol: Alcohol intake during pregnancy may induce fetal alcohol syndrome, leading to developmental delays and ongoing issues.
Addressing any concerns or questions regarding dietary limitations with a healthcare physician is vital.

6.3 Keeping hydrated during exercise

Keeping hydrated while exercising is vital for everyone but particularly critical for pregnant women. Dehydration may lead to complications such as premature delivery, urinary tract infections, and low amniotic fluid levels. Consequently, drinking enough water before, during, and after exercise is crucial.

The American Academy of Obstetricians and Gynecologists (ACOG) advises that pregnant women drink at least 8-12 cups of water daily. However, this quantity may need to be increased during activity. Consuming around 17-20 ounces of water 2-3 hours before a workout and then 7-10 ounces every 10-20 minutes throughout exercise is advisable.

If you are engaged in high-intensity or long-duration activity, consider consuming a sports drink with electrolytes to help restore the minerals lost via sweat. Nonetheless, speaking with your healthcare physician before drinking sports drinks or other supplements during pregnancy is vital.

In addition to water and sports drinks, additional hydration alternatives include coconut water, fruit-infused water, and herbal teas. It is vital to avoid heavy sugar or caffeine liquids, such as soda, coffee, and energy drinks, since these may contribute to dehydration.

Overall, keeping hydrated during activity is vital for the mother's and growing fetus's health and well-being. Be careful to speak to your healthcare practitioner about your particular hydration requirements during pregnancy, and add frequent water breaks into your activity regimen.

Chapter Seven

7.0 Dealing with Common Pregnancy-Related Discomforts

Pregnancy is a joyful experience but may also come with its fair share of discomforts. Pregnancy may bring discomfort in many ways, from morning sickness to back pain. Yet, numerous strategies exist to deal with these discomforts and make the experience more tolerable. Here are some strategies for dealing with typical pregnancy-related pains:

Nausea and vomiting: Many women have morning sicknesses during the first trimester of pregnancy. To deal with this pain, eating small, frequent meals throughout the day is recommended, such as avoiding spicy or oily foods and drinking lots of fluids. Some women get comfort from ginger or vitamin B6 pills or acupressure bands.

Back pain: When the uterus expands, it may exert tension on the back muscles, resulting in discomfort. To deal with this, strive to keep excellent posture, avoid lifting heavy things, wear supportive shoes, and utilize pillows for support when sleeping.

Fatigue: Pregnancy may produce weariness owing to hormonal changes and increasing physical demands on the body. To deal with this, get enough rest, nap during the day, and emphasize sleep at night.

Constipation: Hormonal changes and the growing uterus can slow digestion, leading to constipation. To cope with this, drink plenty of fluids, eat fiber-rich foods such as fruits, vegetables, and whole grains, and exercise regularly.

Heartburn: As the uterus expands, it can push the stomach upwards, leading to heartburn. To cope with this, eat small, frequent meals throughout the day, avoid spicy or greasy foods, and avoid lying down immediately after eating.

Swelling: During pregnancy, the body retains more fluid, leading to swelling in the legs and ankles. To cope with this, elevate your feet when sitting or lying down, avoid standing or sitting for prolonged periods, wear supportive stockings, and exercise regularly.

Mood changes: Hormonal changes during pregnancy can lead to mood swings and emotional distress. To cope with this, practice relaxation techniques such as meditation or yoga, talk to a trusted friend or therapist and engage in activities that bring you joy.

It is important to note that if any discomforts become severe or persistent, it is best to seek medical advice from a healthcare provider. Pregnancy may be a more pleasant and joyful experience with good self-care and medical attention.

7.1 Nausea and vomiting

Nausea and vomiting are frequent discomforts experienced by many pregnant women, especially during the first trimester. It is assumed to be caused by the hormonal changes that occur during pregnancy, specifically the elevated levels of the hormone human chorionic gonadotropin (hCG)

To deal with nausea and vomiting during pregnancy, it is advisable to consume small, frequent meals throughout the day to help maintain blood sugar levels consistent. It is also advised to avoid foods or smells that trigger nausea and to eat bland, low-fat foods such as crackers, rice, or bananas. Drinking fluids, particularly water and ginger tea, can also help alleviate symptoms.

Some women may benefit from taking vitamin B6 supplements or anti-nausea medications prescribed by their healthcare provider. Acupressure, acupuncture, and hypnosis may also be helpful for some women.

It is important to note that while nausea and vomiting can be uncomfortable, they usually do not pose a risk to the mother's or baby's health. However, severe or persistent vomiting may lead to dehydration or weight loss, which can be concerning and require medical attention.

7.2 Fatigue

Fatigue is a joint discomfort experienced during pregnancy, especially during the first and third trimesters. Hormonal changes, increased physical demands on the body, and difficulty sleeping can cause it.

To cope with fatigue, it's important to prioritize rest and relaxation. This may entail taking naps during the day or altering your sleep routine to ensure you're receiving adequate rest at night. Splitting your everyday activities into more minor, manageable chores and preventing overexerting yourself is also good.

Keeping a balanced diet and staying hydrated may also help battle weariness. Consuming a balanced diet with enough fruits, vegetables, and protein helps give the body the nutrients it needs to operate efficiently. Drinking adequate water and avoiding coffee and alcohol helps keep you energetic.

Lastly, exercise may be suitable for lowering weariness during pregnancy. Although it may seem paradoxical, low to moderate exercise may raise energy levels and enhance sleep quality. But, talking with your healthcare professional before initiating any new workout regimen during pregnancy is vital.

7.3 Backache

Back pain is a frequent problem experienced by many pregnant women, particularly during the second and third trimesters. The weight increase and postural changes during pregnancy may stress the back muscles, producing pain and discomfort. Here are some ideas for managing back hurt during pregnancy:

Practice excellent posture: Keeping a good posture might help relieve back discomfort. Stand up straight, with your shoulders back and relaxed, and avoid slouching. While sitting, pick a chair with adequate back support, or use a small cushion to support your lower back.

Exercise: Regular exercise can help strengthen the muscles in your back and abdomen, which can help reduce back pain. Walking, swimming, and prenatal yoga are all healthy alternatives for pregnant women.

Choose the correct shoes: Wearing shoes with solid arch support will help alleviate back discomfort. Avoid high heels or shoes with flat bottoms.

Heat or cold therapy: Applying a warm or cold compress to the affected area can help reduce pain and inflammation. A warm bath or shower can also help relax tense muscles.

Obtain frequent prenatal massages: Prenatal massages may help relieve stress in the back muscles and encourage relaxation.

Employ good body mechanics: When lifting something, bend your knees and lift using your legs, not your back. Avoid twisting your body when lifting. Consider a support belt: A maternal support belt may assist in supporting your lower back and ease back strain.

If your back discomfort is severe or accompanied by other symptoms, such as fever or vaginal bleeding, contacting your healthcare practitioner is vital to rule out any significant issues.

7.4 Leg cramps

Leg cramps are a frequent pain experienced by pregnant women, especially during the second and third trimesters. These cramps may vary from minor to severe and commonly originate in the calf muscles but can also affect the thighs and foot.

The specific origin of leg cramps during pregnancy is not established. However, it is considered to be connected to changes in the body's circulation and metabolism. When the uterus expands and strains the blood arteries that send blood from the legs to the heart, blood flow to the legs might become limited. Moreover, hormonal changes and increased muscle stress during pregnancy might also lead to leg cramps.

There are various things that pregnant women may take to assist decrease leg cramps. Keeping hydrated is vital, since dehydration may worsen muscular cramps. Mild stretching activities, such as calf stretches, are also helpful. Applying heat or ice to the afflicted region and gently rubbing the muscle might also bring comfort. Using supportive shoes and avoiding standing or sitting for a long time is also helpful.

If leg cramps are severe or persistent or are accompanied by swelling, redness, or warmth in the afflicted region, it is crucial to seek medical assistance, since these symptoms might be signals of a blood clot.

Chapter Eight

8.0 Preparing for Labor and Delivery Via Exercise

8.1 Strengthening the pelvic floor muscles

The pelvic floor muscles are a set of muscles that support the pelvic organs, including the bladder, uterus, and rectum. During pregnancy, these muscles might weaken due to the extra weight and strain of the developing baby, which can lead to pain, urine incontinence, and other difficulties. Strengthening the pelvic floor muscles can help prevent these problems and improve overall pelvic health.

One of the best ways to strengthen the pelvic floor muscles is through Kegel exercises. Kegels involve contracting and relaxing the pelvic floor muscles repeatedly. To perform Kegels, first, identify the pelvic floor muscles by trying to stop the flow of urine mid-stream. Once you have located the muscles, contract them for about 5 seconds, then relax for 5 seconds. Repeat this ten times, several times a day.

Another exercise that can help strengthen the pelvic floor muscles is the bridge pose. To do the bridge pose:

1. Lie on your back with your knees bent and feet flat on the floor.
2. Lift your hips off the ground, squeezing your buttocks and pelvic floor muscles as you do so.
3. Hold for 5 seconds, then lower back down to the starting position.
4. Repeat this ten times.

It's important to note that not all pelvic floor exercises are appropriate for every stage of pregnancy. Some activities may be more suitable for specific trimesters or may need to be modified as the pregnancy progresses. It's always a good idea to consult a healthcare provider or pelvic floor physical therapist for guidance on which exercises are safe and effective.

8.2 Relaxation techniques

During pregnancy, finding ways to manage stress and promote relaxation for both physical and mental health is essential. Here are some relaxation techniques that may help:

Breathing exercises: Deep breathing exercises can help you calm down and feel more centered. Try breathing in deeply through your nose and slowly exhaling through your mouth. Concentrate on the feeling of the breath going in and out of your body.

Progressive muscle relaxation: This method includes tensing and relaxing various muscle groups, beginning at your toes and working up to your head. Doing this relieves tension and minimizes muscular soreness.

Guided imagery: This approach includes envisioning a serene or relaxing scenario in your mind. You may shut your eyes and visualize yourself in a quiet environment like a beach or forest.

Yoga and meditation: Doing yoga and meditation may help you relax and decrease tension. These routines may also help you keep flexible and limber throughout pregnancy.

Massage: Prenatal massage may help reduce stress and encourage relaxation. Be cautious about locating a massage therapist educated in dealing with pregnant ladies.

Warm bath or shower: Having a warm bath or shower might help you relax and alleviate muscular tension.
It's crucial to listen to your body throughout pregnancy and identify relaxing methods that work

for you. Make time for self-care and prioritize your physical and emotional well-being.

8.2.1 Breathing exercises

Breathing exercises may be beneficial during pregnancy to decrease tension and anxiety, boost oxygen flow to the body, and prepare for labor and delivery. Several kinds of breathing exercises may be undertaken during pregnancy, including:

Belly breathing entails laying one hand on the belly and the other on the chest, taking deep breaths through the nose, filling the stomach with air, and expanding it as much as possible. Exhale through the lips, forcing all the air out from the belly, and engage the muscles in the lower abdomen.

Equal breathing entails inhaling and exhaling for the exact count, such as inhaling for four counts and exhaling for four counts. This helps to produce a feeling of balance and serenity.

Alternating breathing includes shutting one nostril and inhaling through the other, then closing the different nose and exhaling through the first. This helps to balance the left and right sides of the brain and may be especially effective for lowering stress and anxiety.

Breath counting: This entails counting each inhales and exhale up to a specified number, such as 10 or 20, and then beginning again. This helps to concentrate the mind and stop racing thoughts.

Breathing exercises may be performed at any time throughout the day, but practicing them before bed or in the morning can be excellent to start the day on a peaceful note. These may also be included in a yoga or meditation practice. It's crucial to remember to breathe gently and deeply and never to hold your breath during pregnancy.

8.2.2 Progressive muscular relaxation

Progressive muscle relaxation (PMR) is a relaxation method that includes tensing and then releasing various muscle groups in the body. This approach is intended to decrease tension, stress, and anxiety. It is also beneficial for patients with difficulty sleeping or muscular tension due to chronic pain.

The fundamental premise of PMR is to contract a muscle group for roughly 5-10 seconds and then release the tension, enabling the muscle to relax fully. This may be done while laying down or sitting in a comfortable posture. PMR is often done systematically, beginning with the feet and going upward to the head.

Following are the steps to practice PMR:

- Locate a quiet, comfortable area to sit or lay down.
- Take a few deep breaths to help you relax.
- Tension the muscles in your feet by curling your toes downward, holding for 5-10 seconds, and then releasing the pressure.
- Then, contract your calf muscles by pointing your toes toward your knees, hold for 5-10 seconds, and then release the tension.
- Move upward to your thighs, buttocks, abdomen, chest, back, arms, and hands, repeating the process of tensing and relaxing each muscle group.
- Finally, tense the muscles in your face by scrunching up your look, hold for 5-10 seconds, and then release the tension.
- Take a few deep breaths and relax completely.

PMR can be done daily as a way to manage stress and anxiety or as needed to help you relax before bed. It can take a bit of practice to learn how to tense and relax your muscles effectively, so don't worry if it doesn't feel natural at first. Over time, PMR becomes an effective tool for managing stress and improving overall well-being.

Guided imagery is a relaxation method that utilizes imagination to generate a tranquil, relaxing mental picture. This technique is often used as a stress management tool and effectively reduces anxiety, improves sleep, and promotes relaxation.

To practice guided imagery, a person often seeks a quiet, comfortable spot to sit or lie down. They then shut their eyes and begin to concentrate on their breath. Once they are in a relaxed state, they may visualize a peaceful scene, such as a beach or a forest. They may envision this scenario's sights, sounds, and feelings in as much detail as possible, immersing them in the experience.

Guided imagery can be practiced with the help of a trained professional, such as a therapist or a yoga instructor, who can lead the individual through the visualization. It may also be done using audio CDs, books, or applications that give guided visualization exercises.

Research has demonstrated that guided imagery may help decrease stress and anxiety levels, lower blood pressure, and enhance immunological function. It may also assist folks in managing chronic pain and improve their general well-being.

A warm bath or shower may be a simple and effective way to relax and decrease stress during pregnancy. Warm water may help relax tight muscles, enhance circulation, and produce a feeling of serenity. It may also be a beneficial technique to reduce pregnancy-related discomforts such as back pain, leg cramps, and sleeplessness.

To take a warm bath or shower safely during pregnancy, it is crucial to avoid water that is too hot. Experts suggest maintaining the water temperature below 100 degrees Fahrenheit to reduce the danger of overheating or dehydration. Additionally, avoiding soaking in a tub for too long is vital since extended exposure to warm water might lead to dizziness or lightheadedness.

It is also suggested to avoid using any harsh chemicals or scented items in the bath or shower since they may irritate delicate skin or induce an allergic response. Instead, choose soothing, fragrance-free cosmetics that are mainly made for use during pregnancy.

Overall, having a warm bath or shower may be a safe and effective technique to alleviate stress and promote relaxation during pregnancy, as long as you follow the prescribed parameters and listen to your body's demands.

Chapter Nine

9.0 Postpartum Exercise and Recovery

9.1 Resuming exercise after delivery

Resuming exercise after delivery may be a vital step in restoring physical and mental health, but it's essential to do so safely and with the advice of a healthcare expert. Here are some things to bear in mind while beginning exercise after childbirth:

Wait for authorization from your healthcare practitioner: Your healthcare provider may advise you when it is okay to restart exercising after delivery. It is vital to wait until your body has recovered and your healthcare physician has given you the go-light.

Start slowly: Begin with simple activities, such as walking or pelvic floor exercises, and gradually increase the intensity and length of your workouts over time.

Listen to your body: Pay attention to any pain, discomfort, or extreme exhaustion. These might be symptoms of pushing yourself too hard or your body not yet ready for a particular exercise.

Be hydrated: It is crucial to be hydrated before, during, and after exercise. Breastfeeding women may need to consume extra water to keep them hydrated.

Incorporate pelvic floor exercises: Pelvic floor exercises, like Kegels, may assist in strengthening the muscles that support the bladder, uterus, and rectum. These workouts may be done anywhere and at any time.

Consider breastfeeding: Breastfeeding may assist in burning calories and aid in weight reduction. However, it is crucial to eat enough calories to support nursing and activity.

Be patient: After delivery, it might take time to rebuild strength and endurance. It's crucial to be patient and not push oneself too much.

Remember, every woman's postpartum recovery is different, so listening to your body and speaking with your healthcare practitioner before resuming activity is vital.

9.2 Building core strength

Building core strength is a crucial element of postpartum rehabilitation for women. The core muscles assist in maintaining the spine, pelvis, and organs, and they may become weaker during pregnancy and labor. Strengthening the core muscles may assist in improving posture, avoiding back discomfort, and lowering the chance of pelvic floor problems.

Here are some exercises and ideas to help increase core strength postpartum:

Pelvic floor exercises include tightening and releasing the pelvic floor muscles, which support the bladder, uterus, and rectum. Strong pelvic floor muscles may assist in avoiding urine incontinence and enhance sexual performance. To complete these exercises, tense the muscles as though you are preventing the flow of pee, hold for a few seconds, then relax. Repeat many times a day.

Abdominal bracing: This workout includes clenching the abdominal muscles like you are about to be pounded in the stomach. It helps to activate the deep core muscles that support the spine. To complete this exercise, stand or sit straight, exhale, and bring your navel towards your spine; hold for a few seconds, then release. Repeat many times a day.

Plank variations: Plank workouts are an excellent approach to increasing core strength. Start with modified planks, such as the forearm plank, and eventually build up to complete planks. Keep your core engaged throughout the workout to safeguard your back.

Yoga and Pilates: These types of exercise are fantastic for increasing core strength and improving flexibility. Look for postpartum-specific courses or alter postures as required to prevent placing too much strain on the abdominal muscles.

Walking: Walking is a low-impact workout that may assist to enhance core strength and general fitness. Start with short walks and progressively increase the time and effort.

It is vital to start cautiously and listen to your body while increasing core strength postpartum. Give yourself time to heal, and don't push yourself too hard too quickly. Talk to your healthcare physician before beginning any new workout routine.

9.3 Addressing postpartum depression

Postpartum depression is a kind of depression that affects some women after giving birth. Symptoms may vary from moderate to severe and include emotions of melancholy, worry, impatience, and difficulties connecting with the newborn. It is crucial to managing postpartum depression since it may harm both the mother and the infant.

One effective strategy to combat postpartum depression is via exercise. Exercise has been demonstrated to increase mood and lessen symptoms of depression in both men and women. It may also aid with weight reduction, which can be a problem for some new moms.

It is crucial to start with mild exercise and progressively increase intensity and duration as fitness improves. It is also essential to find pleasurable and doable activities with the responsibilities of caring for a new infant. Some possibilities include walking, yoga, swimming, and low-impact aerobics.

In addition to exercising, obtaining expert aid is also crucial. A healthcare physician or therapist may give support, resources, and treatment choices for postpartum depression. Support groups may also help connect with other moms facing similar problems.

It is crucial to realize that postpartum depression is a common ailment, and getting assistance is a show of courage. With the correct aid and self-care, it is possible to overcome postpartum depression and enjoy the pleasures of parenthood.

Chapter Ten
Conclusion

10.1 Recap of the book's significant topics

"Expecting In Shape" is a book that attempts to give counsel and support to expecting women who desire to maintain a healthy lifestyle throughout their pregnancy. The book highlights the need for exercise and a healthy diet and gives ideas on dealing with typical pregnancy-related discomforts and managing postpartum depression.

The book's primary purpose is to urge pregnant women to be active and take care of themselves throughout their pregnancy to have a healthy pregnancy and delivery. The author emphasizes that exercising during pregnancy may aid with weight control, lower the risk of gestational diabetes, and enhance general physical and mental health.

The book also underlines the necessity of a balanced diet, with a concentration of protein, calcium, iron, and folic acid, while avoiding specific items that may be hazardous during pregnancy.

In addition to providing information on nutrition and exercise, the book offers guidance on coping with common pregnancy-related discomforts such as nausea, fatigue, back pain, and leg cramps. It provides relaxation techniques such as breathing exercises, progressive muscle relaxation, and guided imagery.

Finally, the book discusses restarting exercise after delivery and increasing core strength, as well as the need to tackle postpartum depression.

Overall, "Expecting In Shape" offers a thorough guide for expecting women who wish to maintain a healthy lifestyle and remain in shape throughout their pregnancy while also addressing the specific obstacles and discomforts that come with this life stage.

10.2 Encouragement to continue exercising after pregnancy

The book "Expecting in Shape" highlights the significance of maintaining a regular fitness regimen throughout pregnancy and urges women to continue exercising after delivery. The author stresses the advantages of exercise for physical and mental health, including improved cardiovascular health, lower risk of gestational diabetes, higher mood, and better postpartum recovery.

The book also includes recommendations on building a safe and successful fitness plan during pregnancy, considering individual requirements and preferences. It underlines the need to speak with a healthcare physician and seek expert help to ensure safety and efficacy.

Furthermore, the book acknowledges the problems and discomforts of exercising during and after pregnancy and presents techniques for overcoming these hurdles. It includes ideas for keeping motivated, making realistic objectives, and obtaining social support to stay on track.

In summary, "Expecting in Shape" promotes that exercise may have considerable advantages for pregnant women and encourages them to continue exercising after delivery to preserve physical and emotional wellness.